50 TOP GREEN SMOOTHIE RECIPES

For Weight Loss and Detox

EMMA GREEN

Book

7

CONTENTS

FOREWORD

"I love everything about Emma's connection to weight loss and health."

Hi, my name is Nat Lee, and I've spent most of my life looking pretty good and feeling great. That was up until I started eating on the run and allowing my busy life as a mom to take hold of me. While working too.

In truth, I knew I should eat great food, but time constraints and "motherly craziness" got the better of me. I made sure my son ate well. But I didn't, which was silly, really. Parenting is one of those things that just takes over your life, I suppose. So, anyway, I kinda ate loads of stuff I shouldn't, and drank sodas and milkshakes an awful lot. Chocolate and takeout became my best friend, and I became overweight, by anyone's standards. No one really told me I looked bad, I mean, most people aren't that obvious. But when I was diagnosed with a severe illness and bedridden for four years, it became time to do something to help my recovery. I made the change as soon as I could.

Since reading Emma's books, I've lost 18.5 kg (which is 40 amazing pounds). And I've managed to keep it off by following her wonderful advice, and by using her awesome, easy-to-do recipes. I live relatively simply, but her guide to nutrition and her tips and tricks have helped me a bucket load. Thank you Emma, you've literally changed my life!

INTRODUCTION

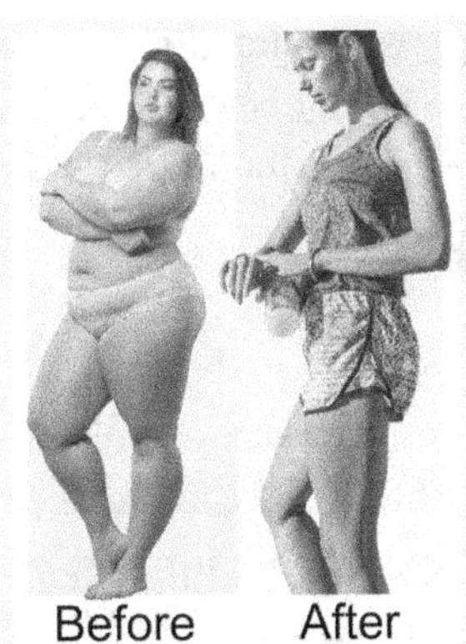

Hi! Thanks so much for joining me here. I am thrilled that you are taking the time to promote and look after your health for weight loss and/or longevity. I want to congratulate you for taking your precious time to read this amazing title and I truly hope you love it!

So, I'm Emma Green, and I live in West Virginia. In all honesty, I lived in a semi-poor family, and we couldn't afford the "right" clothes or any of the expensive cool stuff, and so I was picked on at school and developed social anxiety at a very young age. I ate for comfort, and I guess my problem started when I was around 15 years, or so. This was coupled with the fact that Southerner's diets include loads of big, deep fried foods, barbecues, carb-loaded treats, and a plethora of sugary desserts. Also, because the weather is not as temperate in our state, it's hard to exercise outdoors for most of the year. In reality, it's just too damn hot! And there really aren't that many opportunities for in-state exercises during the months when it's boiling hot, either. On really hot days, it can get up to over 80 degrees Fahrenheit. Our average temperature is around 65 throughout the year.

Please know, if you haven't already read my title, "How I Lost 100 Pounds! My Personal Weight Loss Strategies for Optimum Happiness," make sure you get your FREE copy today. Inside you'll learn exactly how I lost my weight, and the benefits of knowing the must-do nutrition, and other amazing secrets including myths, water weight, cellulite prevention and removal, the only exercise you really need, the ancient and easy technique to help slim you quickly, how to balance meals, and much, much more! I hope you love it. It's my very special gift to you!

It is my hope that you get a wealth of great information from it, and the amazing recipes for both weight loss and detox as well! How exciting! I want you to remember the reason why you came here in the first instance and write down any goals you'd like to achieve. I always find that when you write your goals down, you can have a clear understanding of your "final end goals," and then fill in the bits in-between.

Ask yourself important questions like:

"How can I make this happen in the timeframe allowed?"

"How long will I need to prepare?"

"Will I need to make time for preparation and/or planning?"

Additionally, having a positive mindset is also super-important. I know that I wouldn't be here without that. I actually lost 100 pounds and made sure I stayed positive along the way as a much-needed necessity. Make sure you have a support system (if possible), a really great attitude, and the willingness to push yourself to your end goal/s.

You can totally do this! And I am here 100% backing you all the way. And no matter how long it takes; whether it be weeks, months or even longer!

Let's get stuck in, shall we? Wooo hooo! I know you've got this... yes, you totally do!

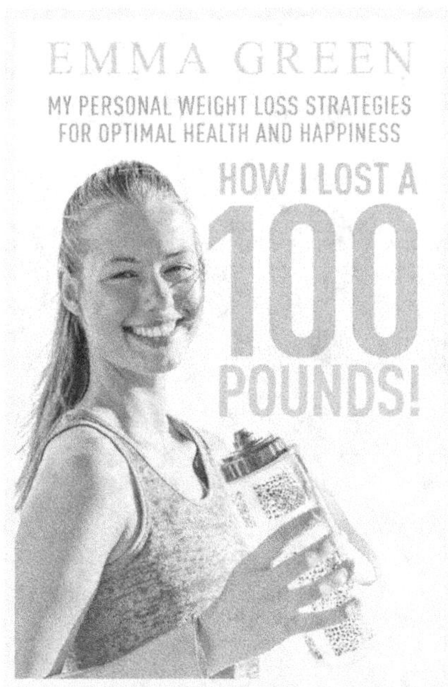

Btw check out "How i lost a 100 pounds" if you haven't already, its got loads of value and its completely FREE :)

FREE GIFTS!

Here are 3 bonus books I want to gift you for coming and reading this title! Sign up to my newsletter and you will receive:

Weight Loss Myths - 9 myths that you are mostly likely doing right now that are totally pointless and are a waste of time toward your weight loss goals.

How to Lose Weight Fast – A 10 day plan I personally put together to make that weight literally melt before your eyes (it worked for me!)

And... Weight Loss Secrets - Secrets the main stream media and health industry never talk about because (let's be honest) things that work don't make them money!

Click here to sign up! or for paperback versions grab it through the ebook completely FREE!

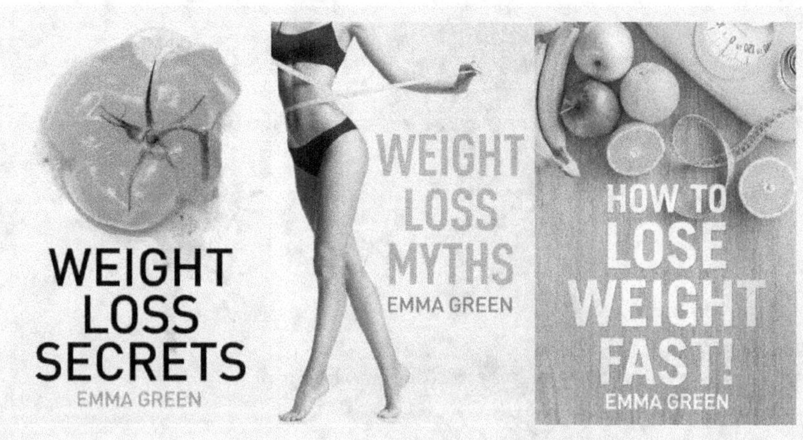

THE HEALTH ISSUES FROM CONVENTIONAL US-BASED DIETS AND THE IMPORTANCE OF ALKALINITY

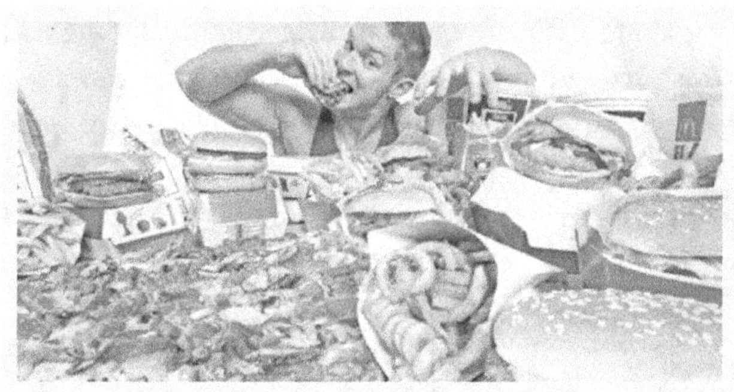

Unfortunately, western-based diets utilize processed foods that are high in salt, sugar, and additives that are not meant for ingestion in the promotion of healthy living. Weight loss is also negated where this "diet" is concerned. From the lack of good diet, and other lifestyle factors (including lack of exercise and stress), the statistics show us that high levels of illness and disease are climbing in the US, and abroad. The high levels are profound and scary, to say the least.

Unhealthy US Statistics:

- Unhealthy diets contribute to 678,000 deaths per year in the US
- Obesity rates have doubled in the US for adults in the past 30 years
- Obesity rates have tripled in the US for children in the past 30 years
- Obesity rates have quadrupled in the US for adolescents in the past 30 years
- Recent reports project that half of all adults will be obese by the year 2030, and that's just in the US alone
- Poor eating habits and lack of physical activity are the top 2 reasons contributing to weight and obesity, globally

It is my hope, that through this book and the expression of knowledge-sharing along with the balance of factors (including adding exercise and stress reduction practices to our lives), we can all spread the word, together. We can also gain insight and see that weight loss is necessary as a vital need for health, as well as for the "feel-good," and "look-good" reasonings that are also important factors in today's society on the whole.

When I look back at all the food I was eating, I was shocked at the way I had been taking nutrition for granted... eventually. Thankfully, I got the right information which helped me to succeed, over time.

It was on a cool summer evening that I was looking online for information on nutrition. I got into a chat page on a website about food. Some of the people discussing nutrition were really awesome. Their knowledgeability just blew me away. They had a lot to say about different foods, and the way they behaved throughout the body. I never really thought about the PH level of food before that night. But, as luck would have it, one guy discussed alkalinity and acidity, and the reason we needed to be aware of it in our own body.

He said something along the lines of, "Hey, has anyone ever noticed how acidic the 'bad foods' are? Most people who get sick or put on weight have a diet that's high in acidic foods."

The comments went on and on down the page, and everyone agreed that this was true. Most obese people (including myself) had diets laden with processed, salty, and sugary foods. I couldn't believe the information could be so simple, and I also learned that we need some acidic foods too. But the balance should be in an 80/20 ratio, of alkaline/acid food. And then our bodies can run in an alkaline state, which is needed for cellular homeostasis (the perfect balance needed for healthy cells and their functioning).

Let's take a look at alkaline foods and acidic foods:

Foods are termed alkaline or acidic depending on what happens to them in your kidneys, essentially. Once the nutrients from the food reach your kidneys, they produce (either) more ammonium which is classed as acidic, or more bicarbonate, which is classed as alkaline. This can be measured and rated, and this score is called the PRAL (Potential Renal Acid Load) by scientists and dieticians.

So, grains, meat, fish, and eggs are considered acidic and have a positive PRAL score. Whereas, fruits and vegetables are considered alkaline and have a negative PRAL score.

In essence, too many acidic foods in your body takes minerals away from your bones which optimize your body's whole PH level.

Some great alkaline foods include: raisins, dates, mushrooms, citrus fruits, tomatoes, spinach, celery, kale, broccoli, and cabbage to name but a few.

All raw foods are better than cooked; you should aim to eat a good percentage of your diet uncooked. This is because when you cook foods you actually reduce the minerals in them that help to stabilize your alkalinity, although, you still will gain the normal vitamin advantage.

Let's take a look at acid forming/anti-alkaline foods:

- **Milk** creates a high acidity in the body and contain carbohydrates, like most **calcium-rich dairy** products.
- **Whole wheat** products, in the form of processed corn or wheat.
- **Eggs**, **lentils**, **soft drinks**, and **coffee** are all high-acidic foods.
- **Peanuts, walnuts, pasta, packaged grain, processed foods, alcohol** and **bread** are also all foods with a high acidic PRAL rating.

As well as the foods we eat, there are other things that can cause high acidity, including alcohol and drug usage (including prescription drugs), a high caffeine intake, artificial sweeteners, stress, excess animal meats, and hormones from foods (health and beauty products). Unfortunately, exposure to many different things can lead to excessive acid build up within the human body.

In most cases, you can utilize the **80/20 rule**. 80% alkaline and 20% acidic, otherwise the acidic PH may cause unwanted symptoms, including illness or a decreased longevity. So, make the change for good, for the benefit of the long term. **Your health is vitally important**. And in addition, weight loss and detoxification can easily be achieved with the incorporation of awesome green smoothies.

THE BENEFITS OF GREEN SMOOTHIES FOR WEIGHT LOSS

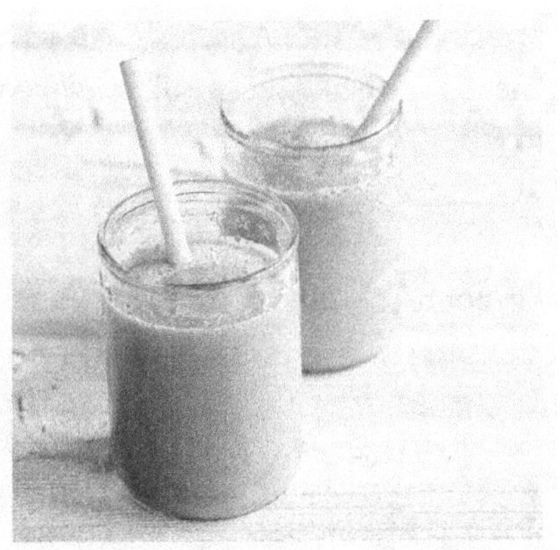

So, when trying to figure out what to eat, it became clear to me that processed, overly salty, overly sugary, and takeout foods were highly acidic. On the no-go list.

On a regular family night, my uncle Harry was talking about the PH of his swimming pool. He added this and that to try and make it perfect. And he was getting to be really great at it too. My aunt was thrilled that he had the mix so good. It didn't sting her eyes, and her hair didn't go green anymore. Thank goodness!

And then I had a light-bulb moment... my cells need to be like a swimming pool! They are made up of liquid that can only come from my drinks and my food. What I eat; they eat, simply speaking.

I laughed at the association, but it helped me to keep it in the forefront of my mind. Each cell is like a tiny swimming pool, needing the love and care from its ingestion of minerals or salts. And to be tended to properly, every day, so it can remain germ free, look good, and function as water in a pool should. No wonder people who don't eat well have so many problems. Their bodies (on the inside) are murky, stagnant, and unable to function at their highest level. This image has stuck with me for a very long time. And it's great to help me remember my cells and their needs. Because after all, they run the entire show! My body...

The alkaline diet (through the use of smoothies) helps to not only get your body's **PH level back to where it should be**, but also to maintain this for the long term.

In essence, your PH level changes from hour to hour, depending on the foods that you eat. The meaning of PH is: Potential of Hydrogen, and this is the measure of acidity or alkalinity within the body. You can use litmus paper to test it.

It is worth noting, that when acidity in the body raises, the levels of minerals fall. So, you could see a level of between 5 and 7 when acidity takes over. **We want to aim for a PH of around 7.4.**

Due to food being mass-industrialized over the last couple of hundred years, food crops now contain less chloride, magnesium, and potassium, with increases in sodium, unfortunately.

If you happen to be vegetarian or vegan, this diet plan can easily work for you because the food contents are nearly all vegetables and fruits. The recipes included have been adapted with weight loss and detoxification in mind. Either way, you can add to them, because they are designed so that they are highly adaptable and useful for variation in tastes, so there is something there that will satisfy your appetite. **Add a nice snack to breakfasts, lunches and dinners**, and make sure your smoothie is the central appeal. I always tell people to make sure they add some meat, fish and protein (like chicken or pork). You want to achieve your goals safely, with health always in the forefront of your mind.

Let's go!!

Chapter One

RECIPE #1: CHIA FREEDOM

Ingredient List:

- 2 oz. of collard greens
- 2 oranges - peeled
- 1 banana - peeled
- 1/4 of a cup of walnuts
- 1 tablespoon of chia seeds
- 1 cup of water
- 1 cup of ice

Directions:

When ready, simply process all the ingredients together in your favorite blender. You can shake it up or stir it up, then serve and enjoy. Cube or chop vegetables to make them blitz easier before blending. I like to add any leafy vegetables in last, and then add a touch more water if I want the consistency smoother or silkier. Great garnishes include: lemon, celery, chia seeds, or a slice of tomato. Add ice on a hot day to make the drink cooler.

Helpful Tips: Adding Rain or Filtered Water

To create a smoother consistency, you can add an inch or two of water. This will create a less dense mixture and will make your juice easier to ingest.

Amazing Facts: Awesome Bananas and Oranges

Bananas and oranges are two of the most familiar smoothie elements, and this is for good reason. They blend beautifully into nearly any recipe and provide a sweetness and creaminess that compliments the savory flavor of the greens. Bananas are full of potassium, and oranges add fiber and vitamin C.

Chapter Two

RECIPE #2: WHEATGRASS WONDER

Ingredient List:

- 1 1/2 oz. of Swiss chard
- 3 kiwis - peeled
- 1 banana - peeled
- 4 tablespoons of almonds
- 1 teaspoon of wheatgrass powder
- 1 cup of water
- 1 cup of ice

Directions:

When ready, simply process all the ingredients together in your favorite blender. You can shake it up or stir it up, then serve and enjoy. Cube or chop vegetables to make them blitz easier before blending. I like to add any leafy vegetables in last, and then add a touch more water if I want the consistency smoother or silkier. Great garnishes include: lemon, celery, chia seeds, or a slice of tomato. Add ice on a hot day to make the drink cooler.

Helpful Tips: Tips to Add in More

Smoothies are awesome because they allow you to add in protein powders and nuts or seeds as well. There is really no limit to what you can add. Go for it as long as it aids your health progression!

Amazing Facts: Wonderful Wheatgrass

One of the first superfoods to gain a lot of popularity was wheatgrass. The beauty of wheatgrass is that it contains chlorophyll, a green pigment in plants that has been shown to support the liver and is well-known to provide a boost of energy, over time.

Chapter Three

RECIPE #3: COCONUT SPINACH WITH PEAR

Ingredient List:

- 1 1/2 oz. of baby spinach
- 2 pears - chopped
- 2 tablespoons of coconut flakes
- 1 tablespoon of hemp seeds
- 1 cup of water
- 1 cup of ice

Directions:

When ready, simply process all the ingredients together in your favorite blender. You can shake it up or stir it up, then serve and enjoy. Cube or chop vegetables to make them blitz easier before blending. I like to add any leafy vegetables in last, and then add a touch more water if I want the consistency smoother or silkier. Great garnishes include: lemon, celery, chia seeds, or a slice of tomato. Add ice on a hot day to make the drink cooler.

Helpful Tips: Blitz the Night Before

Smoothies are fantastic in terms of preparation and ease. You can prepare them in the evening and refrigerate the jug, drinking the blitzed recipe in the morning, and therefore, letting the flavors permeate overnight. If you do this, you won't need to add ice to your recipe, though. Yummy!

Amazing Facts: Coconut Flakes and Hemp Seeds Rock

Coconut flakes and hemp seeds add inflammation-lowering omega-3 fatty acids. Omega-3 is used to help the body lower the risk of heart disease, depression, arthritis, and dementia. Your body can't make omega-3, it needs to be added to the diet.

Chapter Four

RECIPE #4: SUNFLOWER SPINACH

Ingredient List:

- 1 1/2 oz. of baby spinach
- 1 banana - peeled
- 1 tablespoon of sunflower seeds
- 1 teaspoon of cinnamon
- 1 cup of water
- 1 cup of ice

Directions:

When ready, simply process all the ingredients together in your favorite blender. You can shake it up or stir it up, then serve and enjoy. Cube or chop vegetables to make them blitz easier before blending. I like to add any leafy vegetables in last, and then add a touch more water if I want the consistency smoother or silkier. Great garnishes include: lemon, celery, chia seeds, or a slice of tomato. Add ice on a hot day to make the drink cooler.

Helpful Tips: Add a Snack Too

For breakfast and lunch, you can make your favorite smoothie and just add a snack to make it a combo to aid in weight loss. Try grilling fish, or eating a lean pork, chicken or another healthy addition.

Amazing Facts: A Combined Goodness Here

Cinnamon is great as an anti-inflammatory. Spinach is full of vitamins, and the apples add both antioxidants and fiber to the recipe. The banana is great to get potassium and magnesium from, and the sunflower seeds have omega-3s. Wow!

Chapter Five

RECIPE #5: PINEAPPLE-SPINACH FANTASY

Ingredient List:

- 1 1/2 oz. baby spinach
- 4 oz. pineapple - chopped
- 1 persimmon - chopped
- 3 tablespoon of coconut flakes
- 2 tablespoons of dried mulberries
- 1 cup of water
- 1 cup of ice

Directions:

When ready, simply process all the ingredients together in your favorite blender. You can shake it up or stir it up, then serve and enjoy. Cube or chop vegetables to make them blitz easier before blending. I like to add any leafy vegetables in last, and then add a touch more water if I want the consistency smoother or silkier. Great garnishes include: lemon, celery, chia seeds, or a slice of tomato. Add ice on a hot day to make the drink cooler.

Helpful Tips: Top the Persimmons

Take the tops off of the persimmon and the pineapple first, to aid in ease when chopping.

Amazing Facts: Mulberries are Super-Cool

Native to China, mulberries are mildly sweet and contain a very high amount of vitamin C, fiber, and much-needed potassium as well. Additionally, they contain iron, which is needed by the hemoglobin in red blood cells because of its ability to bind with oxygen, and consequently transport it throughout the body.

Chapter Six

RECIPE #6: YUMMY CHAI

Ingredient List:

- 1 1/2 oz. of baby spinach
- 5 oz. of butternut squash
- 1 banana - peeled
- 1/2 teaspoon of chai spice
- 4 tablespoons of almonds
- 1 cup of water
- 1 cup of ice

Directions:

When ready, simply process all the ingredients together in your favorite blender. You can shake it up or stir it up, then serve and enjoy. Cube or chop vegetables to make them blitz easier before blending. I like to add any leafy vegetables in last, and then add a touch more water if I want the consistency smoother or silkier. Great garnishes include: lemon, celery, chia seeds, or a slice of tomato. Add ice on a hot day to make the drink cooler.

Helpful Tips: Keep it Cool or Not

Every smoothie recipe can be iced or left at room temperature if the weather isn't warm enough to drink it cool. The best thing about smoothies is you have so many choices. With flavors, combinations and add-ons! It's only limited by your imagination...

Amazing Facts: Almond Milk and Chai Spices Are Perfect

Almond milk and chai spices create the perfect chai-latte effect. In essence, you have all the flavor of a delicious milkshake with a super-duper nutritional punch.

Chapter Seven

RECIPE #7: PROTEIN GREEN

Ingredient List:

- 1 1/2 oz. baby spinach
- 2 clementine's
- 1 apple - chopped
- 1 tablespoon of flaxseeds
- 1 tablespoon of pea protein
- 1 cup of water
- 1 cup of ice

Directions:

When ready, simply process all the ingredients together in your favorite blender. You can shake it up or stir it up, then serve and enjoy. Cube or chop vegetables to make them blitz easier before blending. I like to add any leafy vegetables in last, and then add a touch more water if I want the consistency smoother or silkier. Great garnishes include: lemon, celery, chia seeds, or a slice of tomato. Add ice on a hot day to make the drink cooler.

Helpful Tips: Take a Sip and Add Organic Honey

Take a sip of your smoothie after it's blitzed. Does it need more sweetness? You can add a tablespoon or two of organic honey to make it sing!

Amazing Facts: Pea Protein and Flaxseeds Accentuate You

With almost 50 percent of your daily vitamin C needs per serving, both your skin and your immune system will thank you for adding pea protein and flaxseeds. A dash of pea protein and the addition of flaxseeds will keep you glowing.

Chapter Eight

RECIPE #8: MINTY GREEN

Ingredient List:

- 1 1/2 oz. of baby spinach
- 4 oz. of pineapple
- 1 apple - chopped
- 1 handful of mint - stemmed
- 1 tablespoon of hemp seeds
- 2 tablespoons of coconut water
- a pinch of sea salt
- 1 cup of ice

Directions:

When ready, simply process all the ingredients together in your favorite blender. You can shake it up or stir it up, then serve and enjoy. Cube or chop vegetables to make them blitz easier before blending. I like to add any leafy vegetables in last, and then add a touch more water if I want the consistency smoother or silkier. Great garnishes include: lemon, celery, chia seeds, or a slice of tomato. Add ice on a hot day to make the drink cooler.

Helpful Tips: Take it to Work

Chill your premade smoothie overnight in the refrigerator. Have one for breakfast and grab another in a drink bottle to have with lunch. You can still be healthy even during the daily grind.

Amazing Facts: Organic Coconut Water is Bliss

Organic coconut water and natural sea salt. When blended with copious amounts of vitamins, your body will stay energized for longer. This low GI recipe is made as an energy booster.

Chapter Nine

RECIPE #9: PUNCHING-BERRY SWISS

Ingredient List:

- 1 1/2 oz. of Swiss chard
- 1 persimmon - topped
- 5 oz. of cantaloupe
- 1 tablespoon of hemp seeds
- 1 cup of berries (amla or seasonal)
- 1 cup water
- 1 cup of ice

Directions:

When ready, simply process all the ingredients together in your favorite blender. You can shake it up or stir it up, then serve and enjoy. Cube or chop vegetables to make them blitz easier before blending. I like to add any leafy vegetables in last, and then add a touch more water if I want the consistency smoother or silkier. Great garnishes include: lemon, celery, chia seeds, or a slice of tomato. Add ice on a hot day to make the drink cooler.

Helpful Tips: Chopping Berries is Good

I like to chop my berries into quarters. The blender can handle whole ones, but it helps the machine to not have to work as hard. We want to do this for a long time so helping the process is always great!

Amazing Facts: Amla Berries Are Crazy-Good

Native to China, amla berries have a long history in Ayurvedic medicine. Full of vitamin C and packed with antioxidants, amla berries have been well-connected to hair health and their ability to lower cholesterol.

Chapter Ten

RECIPE #10: COCONUT SPINACH

Ingredient List:

- 1 1/2 oz. of baby spinach
- 1 banana - peeled
- 1 squash - chopped
- 1 teaspoon of cinnamon
- 4 tablespoons of walnuts
- 1 cup of coconut water
- 1 cup of ice

Directions:

When ready, simply process all the ingredients together in your favorite blender. You can shake it up or stir it up, then serve and enjoy. Cube or chop vegetables to make them blitz easier before blending. I like to add any leafy vegetables in last, and then add a touch more water if I want the consistency smoother or silkier. Great garnishes include: lemon, celery, chia seeds, or a slice of tomato. Add ice on a hot day to make the drink cooler.

Helpful Tips: Plan a Week Ahead

Plan your week of smoothies a week in advance; that way you can be organized when you go to the grocery store. It's super-important to have everything you need to aid your success for the long-term.

Amazing Facts: Jam-Packed with Goodness

This tropical smoothie utilizes great ingredients that taste great and are great for you. With the alkaline ingredient (spinach), the anti-inflammatory ingredient (cinnamon), and the amazing banana; loaded with magnesium and potassium. You can't go wrong with this one!

Chapter Eleven

RECIPE #11: BUTTERNUT-SPINACH SQUASH

Ingredient List:

- 1 1/2 oz. of baby spinach
- 1 banana - peeled
- 4 oz. butternut squash
- 1 teaspoon of matcha powder
- 1 tablespoon of hemp seeds
- 1 cup of water
- 1 cup ice

Directions:

When ready, simply process all the ingredients together in your favorite blender. You can shake it up or stir it up, then serve and enjoy. Cube or chop vegetables to make them blitz easier before blending. I like to add any leafy vegetables in last, and then add a touch more water if I want the consistency smoother or silkier. Great garnishes include: lemon, celery, chia seeds, or a slice of tomato. Add ice on a hot day to make the drink cooler.

Helpful Tips: Your Blender is Important

Blitzing is awesome when you use a good brand of blender/food processor. Make sure you wash it and dry it thoroughly to keep it clean from bacteria and turn it off at the power point when not in use. Remember, kids can put fingers where they don't belong, and other family members too!

Amazing Facts: Matcha Powder is Powerful

Matcha powder is full of l-theanine, a naturally occurring amino acid that helps induce calmness. Great for feeling relaxed, naturally.

Chapter Twelve

RECIPE #12: LUXURY LUCUMA

Ingredient List:

- 1 1/2 oz. of baby spinach
- 1 orange - peeled
- 1 pear - chopped
- 1 teaspoon of lucuma
- 1 tablespoon of chia seeds
- 1 cup of water
- 1 cup of ice

Directions:

When ready, simply process all the ingredients together in your favorite blender. You can shake it up or stir it up, then serve and enjoy. Cube or chop vegetables to make them blitz easier before blending. I like to add any leafy vegetables in last, and then add a touch more water if I want the consistency smoother or silkier. Great garnishes include: lemon, celery, chia seeds, or a slice of tomato. Add ice on a hot day to make the drink cooler.

Helpful Tips: Buy Organic When Possible

A great tip is to buy produce that's organic. That way you are giving your body the best chance at health, by ingesting chemical and pesticide free, (real foods). It might cost a bit more, but the health benefits are worth it in the long run!

Amazing Facts: Lucuma is Like Gold

The Incas of Peru used lucuma so often it became known as "The Gold of the Incas." As well as having beta carotene, lucuma also has the minerals iron and zinc, too.

Chapter Thirteen

RECIPE #13: APPLE PECAN PARADISE

Ingredient List:

- 1 1/2 oz. of baby spinach
- 1 banana - peeled
- 1 container of cinnamon applesauce - (1/2 cup)
- 1 tablespoon of oats
- 3 tablespoons of pecans
- 1 cup of water
- 1 cup of ice

Directions:

When ready, simply process all the ingredients together in your favorite blender. You can shake it up or stir it up, then serve and enjoy. Cube or chop vegetables to make them blitz easier before blending. I like to add any leafy vegetables in last, and then add a touch more water if I want the consistency smoother or silkier. Great garnishes include: lemon, celery, chia seeds, or a slice of tomato. Add ice on a hot day to make the drink cooler.

Helpful Tips: A Smoothie Lifestyle

Once you start having smoothies, you'll notice a change in everything. Your skin, your hair, your weight and even your energy levels. There is no better time to start your weight loss and health journey.

Amazing Facts: Whole Grains, Vitamins and Minerals Needed

A diet high in whole grains like oats helps protect against heart disease and high cholesterol. Banana and spinach provide loads of potassium, magnesium, iron, and vitamin C.

Chapter Fourteen

RECIPE #14: GOJI GO-GO

Ingredient List:

- 1 1/2 oz. of baby spinach
- 1 apple - chopped
- 1 banana - peeled
- 1 tablespoon of goji berries
- 1 tablespoon of flaxseeds
- 1 cup of water
- 1 cup of ice

Directions:

When ready, simply process all the ingredients together in your favorite blender. You can shake it up or stir it up, then serve and enjoy. Cube or chop vegetables to make them blitz easier before blending. I like to add any leafy vegetables in last, and then add a touch more water if I want the consistency smoother or silkier. Great garnishes include: lemon, celery, chia seeds, or a slice of tomato. Add ice on a hot day to make the drink cooler.

Helpful Tips: Eat the Peel It's Good for You

Did you know that eating the peel is great for you? Loads of vitamins and minerals are in the peel. Just wash them well. Do it with carrots, apples, mangoes, pears, and more!

Amazing Facts: Smoothies Are More Than Awesome

Smoothies are great! This recipe utilizes the iron and vitamin K from the spinach, the magnesium from the banana, the antioxidants from the berries, and the omega-3s from the flaxseeds.

Chapter Fifteen

RECIPE #15: PERSIMMON-MINT MAGIC

Ingredient List:

- 1 1/2 oz. of collard greens
- 1 apple - chopped
- 1 persimmon - topped
- 3 sprigs of mint
- 1 teaspoon of matcha tea
- 1 cup of water
- 1 cup of ice

Directions:

When ready, simply process all the ingredients together in your favorite blender. You can shake it up or stir it up, then serve and enjoy. Cube or chop vegetables to make them blitz easier before blending. I like to add any leafy vegetables in last, and then add a touch more water if I want the consistency smoother or silkier. Great garnishes include: lemon, celery, chia seeds, or a slice of tomato. Add ice on a hot day to make the drink cooler.

Helpful Tips: Add More in Experimentation

When you get time, experiment with the recipes and add whatever you like. Maybe a tablespoon of honey for sweetness, another fruit or vegetable type, or something seedy!

Amazing Facts: Persimmons Are Lovely

A great source of both vitamins A and C, persimmons are exceptionally low in fat, but are high in fiber. Giving a really nice boost to your smoothie. Leave the skins on if you want! Wash well and choose organic where possible.

Chapter Sixteen

RECIPE #16: PEARS N' SPINACH

Ingredient List:

- 1 1/2 oz. of baby spinach
- 1 apple - chopped
- 1 pear - chopped
- 1 teaspoon of cinnamon
- 1 tablespoon of flaxseeds
- 1 cup of water
- 1 cup of ice

Directions:

When ready, simply process all the ingredients together in your favorite blender. You can shake it up or stir it up, then serve and enjoy. Cube or chop vegetables to make them blitz easier before blending. I like to add any leafy vegetables in last, and then add a touch more water if I want the consistency smoother or silkier. Great garnishes include: lemon, celery, chia seeds, or a slice of tomato. Add ice on a hot day to make the drink cooler.

Helpful Tips: Use Rainwater, Filtered Water, or Spring Water

It's always important to drink healthy water. We want to limit the chemicals and additives as much as possible... even in our smoothies. Choose rain water, filtered water or spring water.

Amazing Facts: Tasteless Greens Still Give Goodness

A mild green that is routinely tasteless in smoothies is great. Spinach is full of iron, vitamin K, and even more fiber than many other vegetables.

Chapter Seventeen

RECIPE #17: THE LIMEY GRAPE

Ingredient List:

- 1 1/2 oz. of collard greens
- 4 oz. of grapes
- 2 mini cucumbers - chopped
- 1 lime - juiced
- 1 tablespoon of chia seeds
- 1 cup of ice
- 1 cup of water

Directions:

When ready, simply process all the ingredients together in your favorite blender. You can shake it up or stir it up, then serve and enjoy. Cube or chop vegetables to make them blitz easier before blending. I like to add any leafy vegetables in last, and then add a touch more water if I want the consistency smoother or silkier. Great garnishes include: lemon, celery, chia seeds, or a slice of tomato. Add ice on a hot day to make the drink cooler.

Helpful Tips: Coconut Water to Substitute

If you want to add a healthy fat to your smoothie, coconut water is a great way to give your recipe a boost it needs. Swap out the normal water for the coconut water. It's as easy as ABC!

Amazing Facts: Grapes Are Always Amazing

Grapes add a refreshing kick to this smoothie with antioxidants and a touch of sweetness, while curbing sugar cravings and boosting your immunity as well.

Chapter Eighteen

RECIPE #18: ALMOND SCRUMPTIOUS

Ingredient List:

- 1 1/2 oz. of Swiss chard
- 4 oz. of pineapple
- 1 banana - peeled
- 1/2 teaspoon of protein powder
- 1 tablespoon of hemp seed
- 1 cup of almond milk
- a squeeze of lemon
- 1 cup of ice

Directions:

When ready, simply process all the ingredients together in your favorite blender. You can shake it up or stir it up, then serve and enjoy. Cube or chop vegetables to make them blitz easier before blending. I like to add any leafy vegetables in last, and then add a touch more water if I want the consistency smoother or silkier. Great garnishes include: lemon, celery, chia seeds, or a slice of tomato. Add ice on a hot day to make the drink cooler.

Helpful Tips: Alkalize with Tangy Lemon

Although lemons have an acidic taste to them, they actually create an alkalinity within the body. They are great to add in (as a squeeze) or as a garnish you can suck on.

Amazing Facts: Pineapples Rock a Real-Lot

In addition to being rich in vitamin C, pineapples are also bursting with manganese. Manganese is a vital trace mineral that is essential for collagen production, healthy bones and antioxidant defense. It's packed full of fiber too!

Chapter Nineteen

RECIPE #19: APPLE-CUCUMBER SMOOTHIE

Ingredient List:

- 1 1/2 oz. of collard greens
- 1 apple - chopped
- 1 mini cucumber - chopped
- 1 lemon - peeled
- 1/2 an inch of ginger
- 1 tablespoon of sunflower seeds
- 1 cup of water
- 1 cup of ice

Directions:

When ready, simply process all the ingredients together in your favorite blender. You can shake it up or stir it up, then serve and enjoy. Cube or chop vegetables to make them blitz easier before blending. I like to add any leafy vegetables in last, and then add a touch more water if I want the consistency smoother or silkier. Great garnishes include: lemon, celery, chia seeds, or a slice of tomato. Add ice on a hot day to make the drink cooler.

Helpful Tips: Do Smoothies with a Friend

If you love doing stuff in the kitchen, make a day of it with a friend. You can chop and blitz together, experimenting as you go! Then health and friendship can reign.

Amazing Facts: Ginger Is Incredible

Amazingly, ginger is an incredibly warming spice. And in addition to being an anti-inflammatory powerhouse, studies have now shown that regular consumption of ginger may help to burn fat and balance glucose levels within the body.

Chapter Twenty

RECIPE #20: BEAUTIFUL BOK CHOY

Ingredient List:

- 1 1/2 oz. of baby bok choy
- 1 pear – chopped
- 1 banana – sliced
- 1 orange - juiced
- 1 container of cinnamon applesauce - (1/2 cup)
- 1 tablespoon of hemp protein
- 1 tablespoon of sunflower seeds
- 1 cup of water
- 1 cup of ice

Directions:

When ready, simply process all the ingredients together in your favorite blender. You can shake it up or stir it up, then serve and enjoy. Cube or chop vegetables to make them blitz easier before blending. I like to add any leafy vegetables in last, and then add a touch more water if I want the consistency smoother or silkier. Great garnishes include: lemon, celery, chia seeds, or a slice of tomato. Add ice on a hot day to make the drink cooler.

Helpful Tips: Plan on Holiday

Before you go away, write down a list of recipes you will use and try to source the ingredients locally if you can. If you aren't trekking too far from home, then you can take your ingredients with you!

Amazing Facts: Spectacular Sunflower Seeds

Sunflower seeds are beneficial to health because they can help to lower the risk of cardiovascular disease and type 2 diabetes. Rich in vitamin E, vitamin B-1, and copper. I really love sunflower seeds!

Chapter Twenty-One

RECIPE #21: CACTUS CREATION

Ingredient List:

- 1 1/2 oz. of Swiss chard
- 4 oz. pineapple
- 1 banana - peeled
- 1/2 teaspoon of camu powder
- 1 tablespoon of hemp seeds
- 11.5 fl. oz. cactus water
- 1 cup of ice

Directions:

When ready, simply process all the ingredients together in your favorite blender. You can shake it up or stir it up, then serve and enjoy. Cube or chop vegetables to make them blitz easier before blending. I like to add any leafy vegetables in last, and then add a touch more water if I want the consistency smoother or silkier. Great garnishes include: lemon, celery, chia seeds, or a slice of tomato. Add ice on a hot day to make the drink cooler.

Helpful Tips: Separate Bananas

If you separate bananas, you can make them last longer. When they are left joined in a bunch, they tend to brown quicker, which is great if they aren't ripe enough yet.

Amazing Facts: Cactus Water is OMG

Cactus water is highly beneficial to the body. The powerful antioxidants contained inside are known for their rejuvenating and revitalizing benefits to the skin. In addition, there are electrolytes, vitamins, minerals, and it is the only prickly pear cactus fruit containing all 24 betalains (antioxidants).

Chapter Twenty-Two

RECIPE #22: GRAPES N' MORE

Ingredient List:

- 1 1/2 oz. of collard greens
- 4 oz. of grapes
- 1 apple - chopped
- 1 tablespoon of sunflower seeds
- 1 tablespoon of chia seeds
- 1 cup of water
- 1 cup of ice

Directions:

When ready, simply process all the ingredients together in your favorite blender. You can shake it up or stir it up, then serve and enjoy. Cube or chop vegetables to make them blitz easier before blending. I like to add any leafy vegetables in last, and then add a touch more water if I want the consistency smoother or silkier. Great garnishes include: lemon, celery, chia seeds, or a slice of tomato. Add ice on a hot day to make the drink cooler.

Helpful Tips: Add Seeds for More

Any smoothie recipe can be added to. Add seeds like sunflower, hemp, chia, or sesame seeds to the mix. The more goodness the better, that's for sure!

Amazing Facts: Collard Greens Are Stunning

Collard greens are cruciferous vegetables that contain antioxidants and aid in weight loss. They are vital to help alkalize the body, which in turn, helps to maintain the PH needed by cells for homeostasis.

Chapter Twenty-Three

RECIPE #23: GINGER NINJA

Ingredient List:

- 1 1/2 oz. of baby spinach
- 1 apple - chopped
- 2 mini cucumbers - chopped
- 2.5 oz. of lemon ginger
- 2 tablespoons of flaxseeds
- 1 tablespoon of hempseeds
- 1 cup of water (or) coconut water
- 1 cup of ice

Directions:

When ready, simply process all the ingredients together in your favorite blender. You can shake it up or stir it up, then serve and enjoy. Cube or chop vegetables to make them blitz easier before blending. I like to add any leafy vegetables in last, and then add a touch more water if I want the consistency smoother or silkier. Great garnishes include: lemon, celery, chia seeds, or a slice of tomato. Add ice on a hot day to make the drink cooler.

Helpful Tips: Juice for Breakfast, Lunch and Dinner

The great thing about green smoothies is that they can be utilized for each main meal of the day. Add them to a light meal for breakfast, lunch and dinner. You really can't go wrong!

Amazing Facts: Fight Disease with Greens

Greens aid the body because they are high in antioxidants, which help to fight free radical damage within the body. The other awesome thing is that they alkalize the body, helping the individual to create an alkaline PH which is necessary for cellular functioning and healing as a necessity.

Chapter Twenty-Four

RECIPE #24: APPLE-WALNUT WONDERLAND

Ingredient List:

- 1 1/2 oz. of collard greens
- a handful of baby spinach
- 1 orange - peeled
- 1 apple - chopped
- 1 banana
- 3 tablespoons of walnuts
- 1 tablespoon of flaxseeds
- 1 tablespoon of sunflower seeds
- 1 cup of water
- 1 cup of ice

Directions:

When ready, simply process all the ingredients together in your favorite blender. You can shake it up or stir it up, then serve and enjoy. Cube or chop vegetables to make them blitz easier before blending. I like to add any leafy vegetables in last, and then add a touch more water if I want the consistency smoother or silkier. Great garnishes

include: lemon, celery, chia seeds, or a slice of tomato. Add ice on a hot day to make the drink cooler.

Helpful Tips: Add Protein to Aid Nutrition

Protein is found in fish, meat and eggs. Make sure your light meals have some protein in them, that way they'll compliment the smoothies you choose for the day. Awesome stuff!

Amazing Facts: Water Goodness is Beneficial

Adding water to your smoothie is great. The body needs water to help promote weight loss, flush out unwanted toxins, increase energy, relieve fatigue, and to prevent cramps and sprains.

Chapter Twenty-Five

RECIPE #25: KICKSTARTER KIWI

Ingredient List:

- 1 1/2 oz. of baby spinach
- 1 pear - chopped
- 2 kiwis - peeled
- 1 persimmon - chopped
- 1/2 a cup of mulberries
- 1 teaspoon of protein powder
- 3 tablespoons of rolled oats
- 1 cup of water
- 1 cup of ice

Directions:

When ready, simply process all the ingredients together in your favorite blender. You can shake it up or stir it up, then serve and enjoy. Cube or chop vegetables to make them blitz easier before blending. I like to add any leafy vegetables in last, and then add a touch more water if I want the consistency smoother or silkier. Great garnishes include: lemon, celery, chia seeds, or a slice of tomato. Add ice on a hot day to make the drink cooler.

Helpful Tips: Prepare for the Next Day

Before bed, try and write a list of what you want to achieve the next day. This can help with weight loss implementation, exercise goals, smoothie incorporation, organizing meals, and anything else you need done that day!

Amazing Facts: Kiwi Fruit is Pure Magic

Kiwi fruit contains vitamin C and it's also a great source of dietary fiber, folate and other vital minerals. Known as a sleep inducer, it's also great to aid in sleep promotion too!

Chapter Twenty-Six

RECIPE #26: GRAPEY GROPER

Ingredient List:

- 1 1/2 oz. of spinach
- 1 banana
- 5 oz. grapes - stemmed
- 1 tablespoon of hemp seeds
- 1 cup of water
- 1 cup of ice

Directions:

When ready, simply process all the ingredients together in your favorite blender. You can shake it up or stir it up, then serve and enjoy. Cube or chop vegetables to make them blitz easier before blending. I like to add any leafy vegetables in last, and then add a touch more water if I want the consistency smoother or silkier. Great garnishes include: lemon, celery, chia seeds, or a slice of tomato. Add ice on a hot day to make the drink cooler.

Helpful Tips: Add Parsley or Herbs to Accentuate

For more benefits, add parsley and other herbs to your smoothies. It creates an impact with the essential boost to vitamin and mineral addition and will give extra goodness aiding good nutrition and weight loss promotion, too.

Amazing Facts: Parsley Is Vital for Great Health

Parsley is beneficial for its wide variety of nutrients. An excellent source of vitamin K, vitamin C, vitamin A, folate, and iron. It also contains flavonoids and other essential oil components.

Chapter Twenty-Seven

RECIPE #27: CASHEW-CHIA COOLER

Ingredient List:

- 1 1/2 oz. mesclun mix
- 2 kiwis - peeled
- 1 pear - chopped
- 1 persimmon
- 3 tablespoons of cashews
- 1 tablespoons of chia seeds
- 1 cup of water
- 1 cup of ice

Directions:

When ready, simply process all the ingredients together in your favorite blender. You can shake it up or stir it up, then serve and enjoy. Cube or chop vegetables to make them blitz easier before blending. I like to add any leafy vegetables in last, and then add a touch more water if I want the consistency smoother or silkier. Great garnishes include: lemon, celery, chia seeds, or a slice of tomato. Add ice on a hot day to make the drink cooler.

Helpful Tips: Chop Nuts to Help Out

To help blend faster, you can chop your nuts in halves or quarters, or you can buy the nuts chopped for ease of use at the grocery store.

Amazing Facts: Cashews Are Totally Worth It

Cashews contain vitamins E, K and B6. They are also made up of minerals including: copper, phosphorus, iron, zinc, magnesium, and selenium. Cashews also have antioxidant qualities. Wow! Jam-packed full of goodness!

Chapter Twenty-Eight

RECIPE #28: CREAMY COCONUT PINEAPPLE

Ingredient List:

- 1 1/2 oz. of Swiss chard
- 1 banana - peeled
- 4 oz. pineapple
- 1 bunch of mint
- 1 cup of flaxseeds
- 1 tablespoon of pea protein
- 1 teaspoon of acai berry powder
- 1 tablespoon of pumpkin seeds
- 1 container of non-dairy coconut yogurt
- 1/2 cup of water
- 1 cup of ice

Directions:

When ready, simply process all the ingredients together in your favorite blender. You can shake it up or stir it up, then serve and enjoy. Cube or chop vegetables to make them blitz easier before blending. I like to add any leafy vegetables in last, and then add a touch more water if I want the consistency smoother or silkier. Great garnishes

include: lemon, celery, chia seeds, or a slice of tomato. Add ice on a hot day to make the drink cooler.

Helpful Tips: Buy Fresh and Organic

Aiming to buy fresh, organic produce for yourself and your family is highly advisable. That way, you can avoid chemicals and additives that are not helpful for health promotion or weight loss. And that's great for the end goal, right?

Amazing Facts: Flaxseeds Are Fantastic

Flaxseeds are awesome. They contain micronutrients, dietary fiber, manganese, vitamin B1, an essential fatty acid (omega-3), and help with weight loss promotion too!

Chapter Twenty-Nine

RECIPE #29: PROTEIN HIBISCUS

Ingredient List:

- 1 1/2 oz. of Swiss chard
- 1 banana - peeled
- 2 tablespoon of dried hibiscus flowers
- 1 tablespoon of pea protein
- 1 cup of berries (amla or seasonal)
- 1 cup of almond milk
- 1 cup of water

Directions:

When ready, simply process all the ingredients together in your favorite blender. You can shake it up or stir it up, then serve and enjoy. Cube or chop vegetables to make them blitz easier before blending. I like to add any leafy vegetables in last, and then add a touch more water if I want the consistency smoother or silkier. Great garnishes include: lemon, celery, chia seeds, or a slice of tomato. Add ice on a hot day to make the drink cooler.

Helpful Tips: Sip Slowly to Feel Fuller

If you sip your smoothie, you will feel fuller for longer. And this will also help to stave off any cravings in terms of weight loss promotion as well as aiding in great digestion too.

Amazing Facts: Dried Hibiscus Flowers are Amazing

Dried hibiscus flowers are beneficial to aid in health promotion. They contain antioxidants which help to fight free radicals within the body. Additionally, dried hibiscus is known to lower cholesterol, lower blood pressure, help with digestion, aid inflammation issues, and speed up metabolism which is great for aiding weight loss.

Chapter Thirty

RECIPE #30: LIME DELICIOUS

Ingredient List:

- 1 1/2 oz. of baby spinach
- 2 1/2 oz. of grape tomatoes
- 4 oz. pineapple
- 1 banana
- 1 mini cucumber - chopped
- 1 lime - juiced
- 1 tablespoon of flaxseeds
- a pinch of cinnamon
- 1 cup of water
- 1 cup of ice

Directions:

When ready, simply process all the ingredients together in your favorite blender. You can shake it up or stir it up, then serve and enjoy. Cube or chop vegetables to make them blitz easier before blending. I like to add any leafy vegetables in last, and then add a touch more water if I want the consistency smoother or silkier. Great garnishes

include: lemon, celery, chia seeds, or a slice of tomato. Add ice on a hot day to make the drink cooler.

Helpful Tips: A Great Blender Will Last a Long Time

Making the choice to blend smoothies is super! The importance of a great blender/food processor is vitally important. You don't need to purchase the most expensive brand, but it's good to go for quality, so it will last a long time, and work proficiently as well.

Amazing Facts: Cucumber is Cooler-Than-Cool

Cucumber has a huge variety of benefits including: hydration, flushing toxins, nourishing the body with vitamins, giving a skin-friendly supply of minerals, and aiding in weight loss. Yep!

Chapter Thirty-One

RECIPE #31: DELICIOUS APPLE PLUS

Ingredient List:

- 1 1/2 oz. of collard greens
- 1 banana - peeled
- 1 apple - chopped
- 2 tablespoons of almond butter
- 4 tablespoons of rolled oats
- 1 teaspoon of matcha powder
- 1 cup of water
- 1 cup of ice

Directions:

When ready, simply process all the ingredients together in your favorite blender. You can shake it up or stir it up, then serve and enjoy. Cube or chop vegetables to make them blitz easier before blending. I like to add any leafy vegetables in last, and then add a touch more water if I want the consistency smoother or silkier. Great garnishes include: lemon, celery, chia seeds, or a slice of tomato. Add ice on a hot day to make the drink cooler.

Helpful Tips: Let the Kids Learn Too

Teaching your kids how to make green smoothies is awesome! It will keep them entertained and you can play with the recipes to make them your own. Healthy kids are super important!

Amazing Facts: Rolled Oats Are Rockin' It

Rolled oats are a great source of carbohydrates, protein, and fiber. They are known as one of the healthiest foods because of their qualities.

Chapter Thirty-Two

RECIPE #32: HEMP AND CUCUMBER COOLIO

Ingredient List:

- 1 1/2 oz. of collard greens
- 1 apple - chopped
- 2 mini cucumbers - chopped
- 1 lime - juiced
- 1 tablespoon of hemp seeds
- 1 teaspoon of lucuma
- 1 bunch of dill
- 1 cup of water
- 1 cup of ice

Directions:

When ready, simply process all the ingredients together in your favorite blender. You can shake it up or stir it up, then serve and enjoy. Cube or chop vegetables to make them blitz easier before blending. I like to add any leafy vegetables in last, and then add a touch more water if I want the consistency smoother or silkier. Great garnishes include: lemon, celery, chia seeds, or a slice of tomato. Add ice on a hot day to make the drink cooler.

Helpful Tips: Try to Create Your Own Recipes

This is super fun! I love spending the afternoon in the kitchen, especially when I know how healthy my end products will be. Try your hand at creating your very own green smoothies, it's easy and fun!

Amazing Facts: Dill is Delightful

A great source of calcium, manganese and iron. Dill is an antioxidant food that is full of flavonoids which make it a great anti-inflammatory and anti-viral, too.

Chapter Thirty-Three

RECIPE #33: NECTARINE BOOSTER

Ingredient List:

- 1 1/2 oz. of bok choy
- 1 nectarine - pitted
- 6 oz. grapes
- 3 tablespoons of rolled oats
- 1 tablespoon of pea protein
- 1 cup of water
- 1 cup of ice

Directions:

When ready, simply process all the ingredients together in your favorite blender. You can shake it up or stir it up, then serve and enjoy. Cube or chop vegetables to make them blitz easier before blending. I like to add any leafy vegetables in last, and then add a touch more water if I want the consistency smoother or silkier. Great garnishes include: lemon, celery, chia seeds, or a slice of tomato. Add ice on a hot day to make the drink cooler.

Helpful Tips: Aiming for Chlorophyll

The green in vegetables and fruits comes from the pigmentation called chlorophyll. The reason we want it is because of its ability to do these amazing things: fight cancer, improve liver detoxification, speed up wound healing, improve digestion, help with weight control, and protect the skin by keeping it healthy.

Amazing Facts: Bok Choy is Awesome

Bok choy is beneficial in keeping bones healthy and can be used as an aid for blood pressure stabilization. It's also great for the continued promotion of heart health, inflammation prevention, immunity, and aiding the skin to remain healthy, long-term. So good!

Chapter Thirty-Four

RECIPE #34: CUCUMBER CONNECTION

Ingredient List:

- 1 1/2 oz. of Swiss chard
- 2 mini cucumbers - chopped
- 2 tomatillos - husked
- ½ an inch of ginger - chopped
- 1 container applesauce - (1/2 cup)
- 1 lime - juiced
- 4 tablespoons of cashews
- 1 cup of water
- 1 cup of ice

Directions:

When ready, simply process all the ingredients together in your favorite blender. You can shake it up or stir it up, then serve and enjoy. Cube or chop vegetables to make them blitz easier before blending. I like to add any leafy vegetables in last, and then add a touch more water if I want the consistency smoother or silkier. Great garnishes include: lemon, celery, chia seeds, or a slice of tomato. Add ice on a hot day to make the drink cooler.

Helpful Tips: Tell All Your Friends

Tell your friends about the amazing benefits of smoothies. If they want to lose weight or create a healthy lifestyle, then smoothies are definitely the way to go!

Amazing Facts: Magical Swiss Chard

Swiss chard is fantastic for its use as a nutritional powerhouse. It's an excellent source of vitamins K, A and C. It's also packed full of magnesium, potassium, iron, and fiber.

Chapter Thirty-Five

RECIPE #35: JOVIAL JASMINE

Ingredient List:

- 1 1/2 oz. of spinach
- 2 kiwis - peeled
- 1 banana
- 1 nectarine - pitted
- 1 tablespoon of hemp seeds
- 1 tablespoon of flaxseeds
- 2 dates
- 1 cup of berries
- 1 cup of Jasmine green tea
- 1 cup of ice

Directions:

When ready, simply process all the ingredients together in your favorite blender. You can shake it up or stir it up, then serve and enjoy. Cube or chop vegetables to make them blitz easier before blending. I like to add any leafy vegetables in last, and then add a touch more water if I want the consistency smoother or silkier. Great garnishes

include: lemon, celery, chia seeds, or a slice of tomato. Add ice on a hot day to make the drink cooler.

Helpful Tips: Squeeze First to Test It

Squeeze the fruit in the grocery store to check its ripeness and quality. It's easy to do and will help you get the best flavors into your smoothie. You want firm, and not overly squishy. Try and choose organic if you have the option. Obviously, you can't squeeze melon fruit with a hard casing, so look for color and pigment vibrancy on the surface, instead.

Amazing Facts: Marvelous Nectarines

Nectarines are great for weight loss. A medium-sized nectarine only has 60 calories, and the vitamin C is great to aid the immune system. There's also benefits from the vitamin C that are not as well-known, and they include: producing skin, helping to heal scar tissue, and the production of tendons and ligaments.

Chapter Thirty-Six

RECIPE #36: GINGER LEMON ESSENTIAL

Ingredient List:

- 1 1/2 oz. of collard greens
- 3 oz. grape tomatoes
- 2 mini cucumbers - chopped
- 1 lemon - juiced
- 1/2 an inch of ginger - chopped
- 1 tablespoon of chia seeds
- 1 cup of water
- 1 cup of ice

Directions:

When ready, simply process all the ingredients together in your favorite blender. You can shake it up or stir it up, then serve and enjoy. Cube or chop vegetables to make them blitz easier before blending. I like to add any leafy vegetables in last, and then add a touch more water if I want the consistency smoother or silkier. Great garnishes include: lemon, celery, chia seeds, or a slice of tomato. Add ice on a hot day to make the drink cooler.

Helpful Tips: Add A Cooler Pack to Your Lunchbox

If you need to pack your smoothie and snacks for when you're out, let's say to go to work or a picnic, you can add a cooler pack. That way your smoothie and snacks will stay cool for longer, especially in the summertime. If there's a fridge where you are headed, you might not need to do it. They are a super-awesome idea for kids, though.

Amazing Facts: A Wow to Lemons

Lemons are great alkalizers. You can add lemon to your smoothies and to water to help with alkalizing the body. They are powerful health promotors. Aiding in colon health, they have amazing antibacterial properties to help the immune system as well. Other amazing things about lemons: aids weight loss, controls high blood pressure, cures indigestion and constipation, and helps skin to flourish.

Chapter Thirty-Seven

RECIPE #37: COCONUT CRAZY

Ingredient List:

- 1 1/2 oz. of spinach
- 1 nectarine - pitted
- 1 banana - peeled
- 1 tablespoon of pea protein
- 1 teaspoon of lucuma
- 1 tablespoon of flaxseeds
- 1 container of non-dairy coconut yogurt
- 1/2 a cup of water
- 1 cup of ice

Directions:

When ready, simply process all the ingredients together in your favorite blender. You can shake it up or stir it up, then serve and enjoy. Cube or chop vegetables to make them blitz easier before blending. I like to add any leafy vegetables in last, and then add a touch more water if I want the consistency smoother or silkier. Great garnishes include: lemon, celery, chia seeds, or a slice of tomato. Add ice on a hot day to make the drink cooler.

Helpful Tips: Refrigeration Is Important

Make sure your refrigerator is cool enough to keep all your produce free from bacteria and that it's also clean enough for the storage of food. Sometimes we get busy, but your health is so important, so make the effort. Clean it regularly, just like you would yourself.

Amazing Facts: Yummy for Your Tummy - Yogurt

Yogurt is great. Low fat yogurt is always best during detox and/or weight loss. Choose brands that have low sugar and real fruit pieces when you look in the store. Yogurt is great for your digestive tract. It has probiotics (or beneficial bugs) that live in your digestive tract and keep other "bad" microorganisms under control.

Chapter Thirty-Eight

RECIPE #38: PECAN GREEN

Ingredient List:

- 1 handful of spinach
- 2 oranges - peeled
- 1 banana - peeled
- 1 teaspoon of cinnamon
- 2 tablespoons of pecans
- 1 tablespoon of chia seeds
- 1 cup of water
- 1 cup of ice

Directions:

When ready, simply process all the ingredients together in your favorite blender. You can shake it up or stir it up, then serve and enjoy. Cube or chop vegetables to make them blitz easier before blending. I like to add any leafy vegetables in last, and then add a touch more water if I want the consistency smoother or silkier. Great garnishes include: lemon, celery, chia seeds, or a slice of tomato. Add ice on a hot day to make the drink cooler.

Helpful Tips: Stay Positive

Having a healthy mindset is always needed during weight loss and detox. Sometimes, it can be hard to stay on track, but if you stay positive "no matter what," then everything seems far easier to deal with. Talk to a friend, or have a walk, in nature. Sometimes, the simplest things can do the most good.

Amazing Facts: Perfect Pecans

Pecans are super-good. They are packed-full of healthy, unsaturated fat. The good fat! And just a handful of them per day can lower bad cholesterol. How cool is that? They're also full of vitamin A, vitamin B, vitamin E, folic acid, calcium, magnesium, phosphorous and potassium. Unsalted is always best.

Chapter Thirty-Nine

RECIPE #39: COCONUT-PEAR TWIST

Ingredient List:

- 1 1/2 oz. of Swiss chard
- 1 pear - chopped
- 1 orange - peeled
- 1 teaspoon of matcha powder
- 1 teaspoon of lucuma powder
- 2 tablespoons of shredded coconut
- 2 tablespoon of coconut cream
- 1 cup of water
- 1 cup of ice

Directions:

When ready, simply process all the ingredients together in your favorite blender. You can shake it up or stir it up, then serve and enjoy. Cube or chop vegetables to make them blitz easier before blending. I like to add any leafy vegetables in last, and then add a touch more water if I want the consistency smoother or silkier. Great garnishes include: lemon, celery, chia seeds, or a slice of tomato. Add ice on a hot day to make the drink cooler.

Helpful Tips: Meditation and Yoga Can Help

Meditation and yoga are great to aid sleep, stress, weight loss, positivity, and all the other good stuff. When you meditate and/or do yoga, you allow the brain and the body to relax and detoxify too. We want to feel great, nutritionally speaking, and these things can help physically, mentally, and spiritually, as additional factors to boost your whole regime.

Amazing Facts: Coconut Is Definitely Worth It

Coconut has great benefits. You can utilize its water content, or even flake it by grating it over smoothies. Coconut is known to aid blood cholesterol levels and protect against heart disease. What a cool fruit!

Chapter Forty

RECIPE #40: LEMON-MINTY MARVELOUS

Ingredient List:

- 1 bunch of spinach
- 1 apple - chopped
- 1 banana - sliced
- 2 tomatillos - husked
- 1 bunch mint - peeled
- 1 tablespoon of oats
- 1 tablespoon of hemp seeds
- 1 cup of water
- 1 cup of ice

Directions:

When ready, simply process all the ingredients together in your favorite blender. You can shake it up or stir it up, then serve and enjoy. Cube or chop vegetables to make them blitz easier before blending. I like to add any leafy vegetables in last, and then add a touch more water if I want the consistency smoother or silkier. Great garnishes include: lemon, celery, chia seeds, or a slice of tomato. Add ice on a hot day to make the drink cooler.

Helpful Tips: Just Do It

Yep, just do it! What are you waiting for? I'm not just talking about smoothies, either. Is there something that you've been wanting to do for a while? Maybe this is the boost of motivation you need. So, go write that book, or start that business, or even sing that song in the karaoke bar... you can do it! Just do it. You know you can do anything you set your mind on, right?

Amazing Facts: Terrific Tomatillos

Tomatillos are super-cute! The benefits include: a high fiber content, they're packed full of niacin, they're a great source of potassium, and they are loaded with vitamin C, vitamin K, iron, magnesium, phosphorous, and copper. OMG! So good!

Chapter Forty-One

RECIPE #41: MINTED MAGICIAN

Ingredient List:

- 1 1/2 oz. kale
- 1 banana - peeled
- 1 pear - chopped
- 3 sprigs of mint
- 1 cup of berries (amla or seasonal)
- 1 tablespoon of pea protein
- 4 tablespoons of cashews
- 1 cup of water
- 1 cup of ice

Directions:

When ready, simply process all the ingredients together in your favorite blender. You can shake it up or stir it up, then serve and enjoy. Cube or chop vegetables to make them blitz easier before blending. I like to add any leafy vegetables in last, and then add a touch more water if I want the consistency smoother or silkier. Great garnishes include: lemon, celery, chia seeds, or a slice of tomato. Add ice on a hot day to make the drink cooler.

Helpful Tips: Take Your Time

Remember the saying, "Rome wasn't built in a day." I love that. Your body can be Rome - and everything you do to help it adds on and on to the final masterpiece. Yes, the one that it will eventually become. So, be patient. Great works take time!

Amazing Facts: Praise the Pears

Pears are great! They contain antioxidants, flavonoids and are rich in fiber. They also help to promote weight loss, treat diverticulosis, and are great at aiding the prevention of cardiovascular disease, cholesterol buildup, and diabetes. Wow! I am impressed. Oh, they also help with digestion, detoxification, and they are great at fighting free radicals! Sooo good!

Chapter Forty-Two

RECIPE #42: LYCHEE ALMOND SMOOTHIE

Ingredient List:

- 1 1/2 oz. of baby spinach
- 1 pear - chopped
- 1 nectarine - pitted
- 4 lychees - peeled, pitted
- 1/2 a lime - juiced
- 4 tablespoons of almonds
- a pinch of sea salt
- 1 cup of coconut water
- 1 cup of ice

Directions:

When ready, simply process all the ingredients together in your favorite blender. You can shake it up or stir it up, then serve and enjoy. Cube or chop vegetables to make them blitz easier before blending. I like to add any leafy vegetables in last, and then add a touch more water if I want the consistency smoother or silkier. Great garnishes include: lemon, celery, chia seeds, or a slice of tomato. Add ice on a hot day to make the drink cooler.

Helpful Tips: Workout and Move

Having a great exercise regime is important. To aid the body, you can do some light aerobic exercise by walking, for example. If you want to ramp it up a bit, dancing is great, or even aerobics. Remember to stretch, so no injuries occur. Safety is always the best way forward!

Amazing Facts: Go Nuts for Almonds

Almonds are awesome. They actually aid the body in lowering blood sugar levels, and help in reducing blood pressure, lowering cholesterol, reducing hunger pangs, and help to promote weight loss! Yes!

Chapter Forty-Three

RECIPE #43: KALE N' BANANA SPICY

Ingredient List:

- 1 1/2 oz. red kale
- 1 banana - peeled
- 1 nectarine - pitted
- 1 tablespoons of hemp seeds
- 1 tablespoon of pea protein
- 1 teaspoon of chai spice
- 1 cup of almond milk
- 1 cup of ice

Directions:

When ready, simply process all the ingredients together in your favorite blender. You can shake it up or stir it up, then serve and enjoy. Cube or chop vegetables to make them blitz easier before blending. I like to add any leafy vegetables in last, and then add a touch more water if I want the consistency smoother or silkier. Great garnishes include: lemon, celery, chia seeds, or a slice of tomato. Add ice on a hot day to make the drink cooler.

Helpful Tips: Write a Plan to Get Things Done

I find writing out a plan works well: for jobs, smoothie recipes for the week, exercise regimes, or even my free-time "wanna do" list. Yes, this works super-well. I try to put everything into frames of time, and if I don't get something done, I add it to the next day's list.

Amazing Facts: Kale is Crazy-Good

The benefits of kale (apart from its high, antioxidant qualities) include: It has zero fat, it aids digestion processes, it's full of fiber, it's loaded with nutrients and it has loads of vitamins and minerals, including iron and vitamin B6. Kale is also a great source of omega-3 fats.

Chapter Forty-Four

RECIPE #44: TROPICANA TASTY

Ingredient List:

- 1 1/2 oz. of Swiss chard
- 1 banana - peeled
- 2 kiwis - peeled
- 1 tablespoon of pea protein
- 1 tablespoon of flaxseeds
- 1 tablespoon of chia seeds
- 1 cup of water
- 1 cup of ice

Directions:

When ready, simply process all the ingredients together in your favorite blender. You can shake it up or stir it up, then serve and enjoy. Cube or chop vegetables to make them blitz easier before blending. I like to add any leafy vegetables in last, and then add a touch more water if I want the consistency smoother or silkier. Great garnishes include: lemon, celery, chia seeds, or a slice of tomato. Add ice on a hot day to make the drink cooler.

Helpful Tips: Stay Happy and Centered

Staying happy is hard sometimes. But – you can literally fake it until you make it! Say positive affirmations to help. "I feel great, I look amazing, I am healthy, I am doing a great job," are some examples. Remember, happiness really is a state of mind, and eating well will help this happen too! We're on the right track!

Amazing Facts: The Power of Chia Seeds

Chia seeds are fantastic sources of energy. They contain healthy omega-3 fatty acids, carbohydrates, protein, fiber, antioxidants and calcium, too. The word chia means "strength."

Chapter Forty-Five

RECIPE #45: SWEET MANGO DREAMER

Ingredient List:

- 1 1/2 oz. of collard greens
- 1 banana - peeled
- 4 oz. mango
- 4 oz. honeydew
- 1 persimmon - chopped
- 1 tablespoon of dried mulberries
- 1 lime - juiced
- 1 tablespoon of flaxseeds
- 1 cup of water
- 1 cup of ice

Directions:

When ready, simply process all the ingredients together in your favorite blender. You can shake it up or stir it up, then serve and enjoy. Cube or chop vegetables to make them blitz easier before blending. I like to add any leafy vegetables in last, and then add a touch more water if I want the consistency smoother or silkier. Great garnishes

include: lemon, celery, chia seeds, or a slice of tomato. Add ice on a hot day to make the drink cooler.

Helpful Tips: Lose Weight with a Friend

Trying to lose weight is always easier when you add a friend. You can both keep each other happy and motivated to strive for your goals. Stay focused and get busy, together. If you have a partner or spouse, they are there for support, too. Even if it's just a kind word.

Amazing Facts: Happy Honeydew

Honeydew is perfect. It is high in water content and potassium, creating effective blood pressure levels as a necessity. Honeydew also aids collagen production and tissue repair, so it's really great for skin.

Chapter Forty-Six

RECIPE #46: CHIA ORANGE SELECTION

Ingredient List:

- 1 1/2 oz. of Swiss chard
- 1 nectarine - pitted
- 1 orange - peeled
- 1 pineapple - chopped
- 1 tablespoon of chia seeds
- 1 teaspoon of lucuma powder
- a squeeze of lemon
- 1 cup of water
- 1 cup of ice

Directions:

When ready, simply process all the ingredients together in your favorite blender. You can shake it up or stir it up, then serve and enjoy. Cube or chop vegetables to make them blitz easier before blending. I like to add any leafy vegetables in last, and then add a touch more water if I want the consistency smoother or silkier. Great garnishes include: lemon, celery, chia seeds, or a slice of tomato. Add ice on a hot day to make the drink cooler.

Helpful Tips: Have Goals in Mind

What are you striving for? What's the end goal? Is there a timeframe you want to achieve it in? Make a list of goals, and then what you'll need to get there. I know you'll do it. If I can, so can you! This can be done in any are of your life; weight loss or anything! It's only limited by your imagination.

Amazing Facts: Oranges are OMG-Good

Full of vitamin C, oranges boost immunity and give great fiber. They have no fat, cholesterol or sodium. They are also low in calorie content; 85 calories in a medium orange. Great for health and vitality. We love oranges!

Chapter Forty-Seven

RECIPE #47: LEMON AND RHUBARB SMOOTHIE

Ingredient List:

- 1 1/2 oz. of Swiss chard
- 1 apple - chopped
- 1 handful of spinach
- 1 banana
- 1 peach - pitted
- 2 oz. rhubarb stalks (the stalks only - **rhubarb leaves are toxic**)
- 1 teaspoon of cinnamon
- ½ an inch of ginger
- 1/2 lemon - juiced
- 4 tablespoons of walnuts
- 1 cup of water
- 1 cup of ice

Directions:

When ready, simply process all the ingredients together in your favorite blender. You can shake it up or stir it up, then serve and enjoy. Cube or chop vegetables to make them blitz easier before blending. I like to add any leafy vegetables in last, and then add a touch more water if I want the consistency smoother or silkier. Great garnishes include: lemon, celery, chia seeds, or a slice of tomato. Add ice on a hot day to make the drink cooler.

Helpful Tips: Keep Going and Take a Break

We all have rough days. We might get tired, frustrated, and we can even feel a bit "over it," at times. Take some time out for you and watch a movie, listen to music, or do a meditation (or practice yoga) when you can. You'll feel better soon, and then you can keep going. I believe in you!

Amazing Facts: Rhubarb – Remember, Stalks Only

The leaves are toxic because they contain high levels of oxalic acid. Rhubarb stalks benefit the body by being a real superfood. Rhubarb supports bone health and is rich in fiber, thus helping to reduce blood cholesterol levels.

Chapter Forty-Eight

RECIPE #48: CHAMOMILE APPLE

Ingredient List:

- 1 1/2 oz. baby bok choy
- 1 peach - pitted
- 2 apples - chopped
- 1 tablespoon of chamomile
- 3 tablespoons of cashews
- 2 tablespoons of coconut flakes
- 2 tablespoons of hemp seeds
- 1 cup of water
- 1 cup of ice

Directions:

When ready, simply process all the ingredients together in your favorite blender. You can shake it up or stir it up, then serve and enjoy. Cube or chop vegetables to make them blitz easier before blending. I like to add any leafy vegetables in last, and then add a touch more water if I want the consistency smoother or silkier. Great garnishes include: lemon, celery, chia seeds, or a slice of tomato. Add ice on a hot day to make the drink cooler.

Helpful Tips: Get Enough Sleep Please

Sleep is important because our bodies heal and repair during that time. Make sure you turn off any electronics and keep your temperature cool enough to promote relaxation. We are trying to gain health, and sleep is an important factor.

Amazing Facts: Beautiful Chamomile for Weight Loss

Chamomile is a wonderful herb for health. It's crucial in weight loss and fights tummy bloating as well. Drinking chamomile before a meal is said to promote the stimulation of gastric juices, helping to aid in the promotion of real weight loss. Oh yeah!

Chapter Forty-Nine

RECIPE #49: TANGY MANGO TWIST

Ingredient List:

- 1 1/2 oz. of Swiss chard
- 1 banana - peeled
- 1 mango - peeled, pitted
- 4 oz. of cherry tomatoes
- 1/2 lime - juiced
- 1 tablespoon of flaxseeds
- 4 tablespoons of almonds
- 1 teaspoon of wheatgrass powder
- 1 cup of water
- 1 cup of ice

Directions:

When ready, simply process all the ingredients together in your favorite blender. You can shake it up or stir it up, then serve and enjoy. Cube or chop vegetables to make them blitz easier before blending. I like to add any leafy vegetables in last, and then add a touch more water if I want the consistency smoother or silkier. Great garnishes

include: lemon, celery, chia seeds, or a slice of tomato. Add ice on a hot day to make the drink cooler.

Helpful Tips: You Are What You Eat

This fun saying is quite-literally true. What you eat is what you are made up of – so eat well. A simple but true statement. Food for thought...

Amazing Facts: The Perfection of Tomatoes

Tomatoes are awesome because they contain loads of antioxidants which help to prevent cancer and other diseases. They also prevent bone loss, diabetes, kidney stones, stroke, heart attack, and obesity. Perfect!

Chapter Fifty

RECIPE #50: PEACHY COMBO

Ingredient List:

- 1 1/2 oz. of baby spinach
- 1 banana - chopped
- 2 oranges - juiced
- 1 peach - pitted
- 2 oz. of blackberries
- 2 tomatillos - husked
- 1/2 a lemon - juiced
- 1 tablespoon of flaxseeds
- 1 cup of water
- 1 cup of ice

Directions:

When ready, simply process all the ingredients together in your favorite blender. You can shake it up or stir it up, then serve and enjoy. Cube or chop vegetables to make them blitz easier before blending. I like to add any leafy vegetables in last, and then add a touch more water if I want the consistency smoother or silkier. Great garnishes

include: lemon, celery, chia seeds, or a slice of tomato. Add ice on a hot day to make the drink cooler.

Helpful Tips: Believe in Yourself

You are your own best friend... no one else will care for you like you will. So, give yourself great health by eating well, doing some exercise, staying positive, and remaining as stress free as possible. You are totally worth it!

Amazing Facts: Baby Spinach is a Superfood

Baby spinach is full of iron and other great nutrients. It has great antioxidant qualities and boosts energy too. If you can eat a superfood every day, then your health can easily be maintained... I add baby spinach to everything! Yummy as!

IN CONCLUSION

In Conclusion

So, my friend Jeremy came over to watch a movie on a Sunday night. This was right after I'd discovered green smoothies (of course). He was drinking a soda when he arrived, and I grabbed the can from his hand and said, "Not on my watch!"

He looked at me and rolled his eyes (as he does so well). He said," Oh, here we go... what deliciously nutritious thing do I have to try tonight!" I laughed at his words that were full of sarcasm, and while he chose the movie, I made him a green smoothie. I just made it up as I went along. When I took it to him, his faced turned up as if to say, "Ugh!" He took a big slurp through the straw and said, "Oh my God!" I laughed. He said, "Emma, it's actually really, really, really... good. I got to pick the movie that night... ha! So good. I think it was Twilight. He hates vampire movies! That was the best night! He makes me make them all the time, now. Except he picks the movies... I'm not allowed!

Thanks so much for joining me here, I hope you enjoyed your time with me! I hope you love all of the smoothie recipes as much as I have loved sharing them all with you! Just remember, you can change them or add to them, putting your very own twist on them as you wish.

I know how hard it is to lose weight, and I am speaking from experience when I tell you that it is definitely possible, especially when you know how to do it properly, and safely. Using smoothies as a filler to aid breakfasts, lunches and dinners is the best option to help with a long-term goal for effective weight loss achievability.

I want you to be proud of yourself for taking the journey of weight loss into your hands. Just remember the importance of alkalinity as a necessity to keep your PH alkalized at 7.4. You can purchase lickable litmus paper to test this. When you stay at a level of around 7.4, the cells can then enjoy a level that's perfect for homeostasis (the perfect balance for functioning and replication processes).

Just remember, I am always here cheering you on and I know you can do this! When you have a positive mindset... anything, yes; absolutely anything is possible!

I am sending you all of my love and light on your health and weight loss journey, and I thank you again for joining me here!

Love and light always, *Emma xx*

P.S. Remember, if you haven't already read my title, "How I Lost 100 Pounds! My Personal Weight Loss Strategies for Optimum Happiness," make sure you get your FREE copy today. Inside you'll learn exactly how I lost my weight, and the benefits of knowing the must-do nutrition, and other amazing secrets including myths, water weight, cellulite prevention and removal, the only exercise you really need, the ancient and easy technique to help slim you quickly, how to balance meals, and much, much more! I hope you love it. It's my very special gift to you! I think you'll absolutely love it!

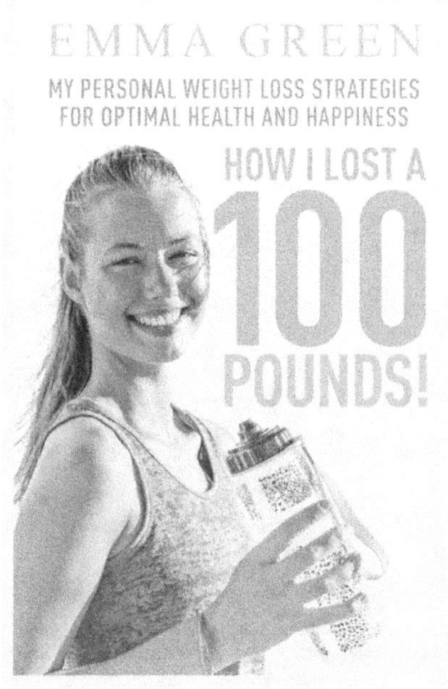

Click here to get your FREE copy or checkout my author profile for more free titles.